MW01602604

UNCOMMON SENSE

A GEN X TALE AND AN INSPIRATIONAL GUIDE
TO ADVOCATE FOR YOURSELF

David Albert Francoeur

Copyright © 2024 David Albert Francoeur
All rights reserved
First Edition

NEWMAN SPRINGS PUBLISHING
320 Broad Street
Red Bank, NJ 07701

First originally published by Newman Springs Publishing 2024

ISBN 979-8-89308-220-3 (Paperback)
ISBN 979-8-89308-221-0 (Digital)

Printed in the United States of America

I thought a lot about what kind of dedication I would want to submit here, and, of course, I have a number of friends and family that I would want to cite. However, I want to do something different. I want to dedicate this book not just to my best friend, my most trusted confidant in my life, but I want to boldly alert you to the fact that this most trusted best friend is also *your* best friend. How so? I dedicate this book to my best friend, my God, my Lord, and my Healer, Almighty God. Dear reader, I know that might sound corny, but please, take it from me. I have spent the past three years battling fatal brain cancer, and I can attest firsthand that, as I did, and everyone can do in life, it is not just highly worth it; it is absolutely everything that you find God in your life. This book is dedicated to injecting greater harmony and good, positive results into our world today with the help of God. Take some time to reflect upon God in your life, and you will unlock your future. Take care and God bless.

Kind regards,
David

CONTENTS

CHAPTER 1

Common Sense and Uncommon Sense

A LONG TIME AGO, A BOOK CALLED *Common Sense* was written by Thomas Paine and published on January 10, 1776. The book you are now reading, *Uncommon Sense*, was formally completed on January 10, 2024, exactly 248 years later. Despite this large time gap, there are many connections between these two books, and that's just one aspect of this incredibly unique story. Both books seek, at their core, to promote harmony amid a backdrop of crazy and turbulent times while presenting some of the most pressing issues of our day in plain English.

Another seismic similarity between these two books is that each author wrote each book, *Common Sense* in 1776 and *Uncommon Sense* in 2024, just after each author successfully overcame a sudden and life-threatening medical illness! And this is a book about how one man overcame sudden, life-threatening brain cancer. These illnesses, smallpox in 1775 and brain cancer in 2024, respectively, almost killed each man. Still, upon "awakening into the world again," both men felt a profound sense of relief and a social obligation to write, write, write their books. As you will read in this book, dear reader, I overcame near-fatal brain cancer—called glioblastoma—the same brain cancer, incidentally, that killed Senator Ted Kennedy and Presidential Candidate John McCain. Because of this, I was heavily influenced by a multitude of immediate real-life experiences that coincided with me receiving the highest levels and dosages of radiation and chemotherapy treatments. This is a book that details my own assertive approach to overcoming this fatal cancer, as well as explaining what were the first healthy steps I took as I reentered our world.

Another seismic aspect of this experience was the extent to which I thought, felt, and believed that God stayed very close to me. In fact, as you will see by my stories that follow, God spoke to me frequently and directly. I provide detail in the following words, but my experience was that God kept telling me to "look, listen, and learn" by all that he wanted to reveal to me. I know it might sound hard to believe, but as I have read many stories of other people who experienced near-death experiences, I think when you read this story, you will understand more about what I really mean. While much of what God wanted to reveal to me dealt with my personal life, it is inextricably linked to revelations that I believe he wanted to share with me about our society as a whole, again, very similar, I think, to the same process Thomas Paine went through in 1775/1776.

My name is David Albert Francoeur, and I am the author of *Uncommon Sense*. I am a fifty-seven-year-old American male whose death, my death, was continuously put in front of me for several months as my doctors gave me their fatal diagnosis and told me, politely but bluntly, that I was going to die and that the statistics for my brain cancer stated that it was likely that I would die fairly quickly. Yikes! But as I grappled with the enormity of what my doctors were telling me, I really heard God speaking to me in many ways. Let me just get to it and tell you now, just what happened!

CHAPTER 2

Diagnosis Brain Cancer

HERE WE GO: BEGINNING IN 2021, DAVID was diagnosed with an aggressive brain tumor and fatal *glioblastoma* brain cancer. David was told many times that he was going to die. I am this person.

I am David, whose book you are now reading, and I am going to switch to my own first-person voice now to continue writing. But first, here is some amazing good news! It is now January 10, 2024, and I am cancer-free. I've been cancer-free for more than two years, and my doctors tell me I am doing *exceptionally well!* Thank you, God. I am grateful. Dear reader, this book you are reading is not just an ordinary book; it is something unique and special, although I'm not going to attempt to explain that. Just read it, and I hope you will find it interesting, maybe even inspiring, and, more so, I hope you will derive some real, tangible value from it for yourself. It's that kind of book. May God bless you. Thank you for reading what I have to say.

The best way to get into the main content of this book is to first explain what happened to me immediately upon learning that I had brain cancer. Dear reader, as you may also know, for people who have confronted cancer or any other deadly disease: the news hits you hard. It hit me hard, very hard. In fact, I am, first and foremost, extremely thankful and grateful to God, Jesus, and the Divine Universe for giving me the strength and the capabilities to defeat this cancer and to now have the great fortune to connect with you, dear reader, by writing this book. Let's get started:

All this first started for me in 2020 when I went out to dinner on a date. While we were having dinner, I excused myself to go to the bathroom. In this restaurant, we were dining on the second floor of a large building in downtown Boston, Massachusetts. I had to walk down a large flight of stairs to get to the bathroom on the first floor. Sounds simple, right? But as I walked down the stairs, I noticed that no matter how hard I tried, I could not walk downstairs without tripping. I didn't think too much of it at the time, but a few days later, I had an appointment for my annual physical with my primary care doctor. I shared with my doctor how I wasn't able to walk downstairs, and he told me he wanted to run some tests. He did, and then he said, "You know, David, something's not right here. We think there may be something neurological going on. We think you should check into the neurology department at any of the large Boston hospitals, explain what happened, and see if they want to run additional tests."

At this early stage in my story, I wasn't really feeling much emotion. I just took everything in stride, and even though my primary care doctor recommended that I consult with neurologists, to me, this was just another errand I had to do. I wasn't feeling anything emotionally.

CHAPTER 3

Hard-Wired to Work

I DID AS MY PRIMARY CARE DOCTOR suggested, and a few days later, I found myself in a prominent, world-renowned major Boston hospital. They had assembled a group of two or three neurologists and a few nurses into a large conference room. They asked me to come in, and one of the neurologists said, "David, look. We ran some tests, and here's the deal. You have a small but aggressive brain tumor, and you also have brain cancer." He continued by saying, "All we can do is give you ten weeks of radiation and then six to eight weeks of chemotherapy, after which time, you will be cancer-free for forty-five days, and then we think you are going to die!"

Whoa! Now I consider myself very much to be a reasonable and nice guy, but think about how you might react if a highly respected neurologist just told you that you were going to die. Within a microsecond of him telling me that I was going to die, I was seriously angry with him for saying that! Again, I am a reasonable and nice guy, but at that moment, I really wanted to punch this doctor in the face! I could feel this emotion boiling up inside of me.

I thought to myself, "We haven't even done anything yet to treat me! You haven't even done any work, and yet, here you are being negative, saying that I'm going to die!" His comments went completely against how I am hard-wired, which is to first work, work, work, and to be positive that you can "fix it." I believe it is something of a sin to be negative, especially if you haven't even started to work on fixing any given problem. I also believe you should force yourself, if necessary, to be positive. You certainly don't start out by being a whiny ass baby by being negative. Period.

Now years later, I respect that this doctor was probably just trying to do a difficult job, but at the time, I was ripping angry. So as soon as he said I was going to die, I put my hand up in the air in the conference room and spoke up loudly so everyone could hear me, and I said, "Excuse me, excuse me, but did everyone hear what he just said? Did everyone hear what this doctor just said?"

Everyone in the room nodded and said, "Yes, we heard him," to which I then turned to the doctor who had just said this, and I said, "I bring this up, and I ask everyone because I want to tell you straight up: 'You're wrong. That's not what's going to happen. I'm going to beat this.'"

The neurologist said, "David, David, look. I've been treating this disease for twenty-five years and, in all that time of treating many, many patients, only a very small handful, so virtually no one, has ever survived this diagnosis." He continued, "This is the same brain cancer that killed Ted Kennedy and John McCain. It's called glioblastoma, and I know what I'm talking about. I'm sorry."

As I said, this news hit me hard, but I am an exceptionally determined person and a chronic optimist. From my perspective, this doctor was violating the first rule of how to confront any serious challenge; he was voicing negativity and not discussing how we were going to fix it. And so behaving somewhat forcefully, I again looked everyone in the room in the eye as I said to this doctor, "You just told me that some people did, in fact, beat this disease, right?"

"Yes," he said.

"Okay," I replied. "Then I want to discuss right now in detail everything you did to treat those people, and then I want to define a program where we do more to treat me." But I still didn't get the type of action-oriented, positive response I wanted, so I kept pushing and said, "You say I have a small brain tumor, so it seems to me, if I have a tumor, that tumor shouldn't be inside my head, right? I would think we should do a brain surgery to remove it, am I right?"

Initially, the doctors all said, "Yes, we should do brain surgery to remove it." Then they all started explaining to me why they felt we should "give it a few months" before they did the brain surgery. I remember I was quickly losing patience.

"No, I don't want to delay the brain surgery for a few months," I said abruptly. "I want the brain surgery right now."

I remember they were not pleased with how abrupt I was being. I started thinking, "Gee, David, you just got some very serious news, and all these guys are very smart and highly respected neurologists. You're not a neurologist. Maybe you should just listen to them?" But then, as if erupting from my inner core, I told them again, "I don't want to delay. I want the surgery right now, tonight."

Their facial expressions told me that I was upsetting them, and as soon as I felt I was pushing too hard, the following thought flashed in my head, "Now you're on point!" Being "on point" is a military term. It stands for being the very front man in your unit directly facing the enemy. You're out front, taking the most risk. It's the most exposed, most vulnerable position. It's dangerous, and this is how I felt as I was aggressively demanding the brain surgery in direct opposition to what the neurologists were recommending.

I was about to give up when something very strange happened: My mind played a trick on me. A memory from when I was ten years old burst into my mind. It presented itself after forty-five years of not thinking about it whatsoever. It came back to me with such unrelenting and astonishing force and clarity that it was startling to have it invade my brain so forcefully at the time. I remember thinking that it felt like something God was demanding me to pay attention to. Still, then, as the end of this story shows, it was this memory, ultimately, that gave me the capacity I needed in that moment to keep pushing forward and to obtain the brain surgery that very night. The brain surgeon would later tell me that he thought, with my assertive actions, that I had "just saved my own life!" Wow.

Before I tell you what that memory was, let's have another brief word about the author of *Uncommon Sense*, David Albert Francoeur. I am a hardworking man in his late fifties. My father was a union construction worker and an immigrant. He was an exceptionally blunt and direct, *old-school* kind of guy. I am a first-generation American. I was one of the first in my family to go to college, and after college, I went on to have a strong and successful thirty-five-year career in the corporate world. Like my dad, I am a good carpenter, and I have worked a lot of hard labor, "pick-and-shovel" jobs, as they say. I know what hard physical work is. With this background and my thirty-five-year corporate career experience, I can honestly say there's a lot the white-collar world can learn from the blue-collar world. I think it's worth saying that, if for no other reason, I rarely ever hear that said and it is abundantly true.

I think back to my *old-school* work crewmates—Mario, Tony, and Americo—with whom I worked my toughest "pick-and-shovel" job using jackhammers, hammer and chisel, and asphalt saws, an intensely physically demanding job. These were some of the smartest and most hardworking guys I have ever worked with. I wish we had time for me to really tell you about them, but the bottom line is that these guys were all just salt-of-the-earth-type guys and, as we all shared seats in the cab of a big truck in which we spent countless hours, they all were nonstop and pleasurable talkers! We gabbed a lot, and, hey, why not divert here for one funny story?

On really hot days, especially if we had been working physically hard, we might drive the truck to a nice spot in a park, and then we'd all just fall asleep sitting in the truck. Well, Tony, as I remember, used to hide a large feather in his coat, and when Mario or Americo fell asleep, Tony would stealthily take out his feather and tickle one of their noses. They would get spooked, maybe slap their own face, and abruptly wake up very upset with Tony for tickling their nose with a feather! It was fun, and I can look back now in admiration that, for guys in their sixties at the time, they were all still laughing and joking around.

CHAPTER 4

Push/Push/Push and Don't Take "No" for an Answer

OKAY, SO HERE'S THAT MEMORY I PROMISED to tell you from when I was ten years old, forty-seven years ago! Now this is an important part of this book for you, dear reader, because that memory from when I was ten is still, far and away, the best advice I have ever received in my fifty-seven-year-old life. That's a big deal, and I can tell you that, over the decades, I've shared this advice with numerous other people, especially those who were going through tough personal times. Many of these people later contacted me and told me that they followed this advice and that it really created positive results for them, as it did for me. It's solid, solid advice for anyone and everyone. Let me tell you what it is:

When I was ten years old, my dad, Albert, was a union construction worker, and on the weekends, he used to take me to his construction worksites. One time, again, when I was ten years old, he took me to a construction site, and I was climbing around the staging when I bumped into another construction worker. He was in his sixties but was also big and muscular. He had some tough-guy tattoos and spoke very loudly. In short, he was intimidating, and when he saw me, he immediately called out to my father and said, "Hey, Albert, your kid is here. Do you want me to explain the meaning of life to him?"

My father said, "Yeah, go ahead."

So then this muscular and intimidating guy started to speak to me in his booming, loud voice. He kept pointing his finger at me as he spoke, and I remember being in rapt attention. He said, "Okay, look, kid. Here's the deal." Pointing at me, he continued, "In this world, you decide what you want or what you need. You decide! You don't let other people tell you what you want or what you need! You decide! And then when you know what you want, you go out into the world, and you push/push/push until you get what you want, and you don't take no for an answer. And that, my son, is the meaning of life. You got it?" After he told me that, he said, "Remember, you don't let other people tell you what you want or what you need. You decide!"

So now back to the hospital story in the conference room with the neurologists and nurses. Just when I felt like maybe I shouldn't be pushing so hard, this memory grabbed ahold of me like a bolt of lightning, and at that moment, I felt 100 percent assured that I knew precisely what I wanted: I wanted the brain surgery to remove the brain tumor immediately, with no delay. And I decided, according to this tough guy's advice, that I wasn't going to let anyone else change my mind or tell me what I wanted. Because this was such a unique experience, to have a decades-old memory so forcefully invade my brain, I remember thinking at the time that it felt like God was intervening to help me: I was glued to it. I resolved, then and there, to push/push/push until the doctors agreed with me, and I was not going to accept "no" for an answer. The memory kept pressing me. So I explained to the doctors that, while I heard their reasoning as to why we should delay the brain surgery, I decided that I didn't want to wait a few months. I respectfully but still assertively told them I wanted the brain surgery immediately—that night!

The doctors told me, "No," and I asked them again and again, and they told me "No" and "No" again. Now as I said, I consider myself to be a reasonable and nice man, but I thought to myself, "Am I too reasonable? Am I too nice?"

I felt God was directly intervening because this memory from when I was ten years old kept superseding me, so I kept pushing harder and harder, and I wasn't accepting their "Nos" for an answer. I remember thinking, "Well, if I have to get ugly, then I'll get ugly."

I asked the doctor, "Who's in charge here? Who's the boss?"

The doctor immediately started to tell me that he was the chief of neurosurgery. I quickly cut him off and said, "The reason I'm asking you who the boss is here is because I want to tell you I'm the boss here, not you. I'm making the decisions here, not you."

Then I asked the doctor what felt like ten more times for the surgery, and ten more times, he told me, "No." Finally, he said, "Look, David, even if we wanted to, we can't perform the brain surgery because the brain surgeon isn't even here at the hospital. He's not here!"

I tried my best to show my sternest face. I looked him squarely in the eye and said, "I'm getting exasperated with all this! What is that?" I dramatically pointed. "What is that right there?"

The doctors said, "What? The telephone?"

I said, "Yeah, that's right. It's a telephone. And I want you to pick up that telephone, and you call that brain surgeon right now." I kept speaking: "And when you get him on the phone, I want you to tell him that you don't care where he is or what he's doing. Tell him he needs to get back to the hospital immediately for emergency brain surgery."

So then what happened? It worked. With that final push on my part, they complied! They called the brain surgeon, said what I instructed, and the brain surgeon was now on his way back to the hospital! To think I got this done because of some very sage and blunt advice I got from a very old school and rough kind of guy, a complete stranger when I was just ten years old! What a trick my mind played on me! Or was it God intervening?

Uncommon sense: This story identifies something that I think is happening all across our society today: Situations are presented to the public as big, major problems when, in reality, just like with this surgery, there is no real problem. We know what needs to be done to fix all our challenges, and we have all the tools and competence to do it. We just need to do it! We'll discuss this more later because, in short, I think that this experience that God revealed to me actually revealed how I believe the United States will resolve all its challenges, starting in 2024, and go on to great success.

Also, more value for you, dear reader: I have told this story several times, most recently just a few weeks ago. The person I told it to told it to another person who soon had a medical problem of his own. That person told me that, as he had just heard my story, he took valuable inspiration from it and then just as I did, was able to successfully push/push/push his own doctors to agree to provide him with something he felt he needed, but that they wouldn't commit to. He told me his doctor later thanked him for pushing so hard and said he would be in a much better circumstance for it now!

So as I felt God was requesting me to look, listen, and learn, and as I discovered how other people took this advice and story from me and then produced their own successful outcomes, I realized that maybe this is how God wants to intervene to specifically help you. Please don't think of this as just another book you're reading; please accept my heartfelt goodwill and God's intervention—take some inspiration from it and deploy this same advice in your own life. If done thoughtfully, which you can do, then you are likely, I believe, to produce something truly beneficial and meaningful for yourself. That's why this advice is so good because it's just such common sense! In fact, become the chronic optimist yourself right now, and just accept that there is a great big value for you right here, right now, so take it by thinking about something important to you, something that you really want or really need in your life right now, and then get started to intelligently, respectfully, and assertively push/push/push to get what you want. Have fun with it. Don't take "No" for an answer.

Another note: Years ago, when I gave this advice to a fifty-some-thing-year-old woman, she later called to tell me how whenever she decides what she wants or what she needs now, she told me, "I feel as if I'm already halfway there to obtaining it because I know I'm just going to keep pushing, respectfully, until I accomplish my goal!" So it works. Give it a try, and may God bless you! You *can* do it! You *will* succeed!

CHAPTER 5

Don't Fuck It Up

BACK TO THE STORY: AFTER THEY GOT the brain surgeon to come back to the hospital, they sent me to a hospital room to wait, and after a short time, they sent two nurses into my room. The nurses entered and said, "David, the brain surgeon has arrived. He's getting ready to do your brain surgery. He just wants to know if you have anything you want to say to him before he does your brain surgery?"

I thought for a second, turned my head, and said, "Yeah, tell him I say, 'Don't fuck it up.'"

The nurses said, "What? No, we can't say that."

And again, I pushed and respectfully told them to please tell the surgeon what I said. They told him.

My next memory was waking up in my hospital room the following morning. At this time, the nurses were walking the brain surgeon into my room and introducing him to me. He was all smiles and in a great mood. The surgeon said, "David, last night, we did your brain surgery, and it couldn't have gone any better. We removed 100 percent of the tumor, and everything went perfectly. This was a delicate operation, but, again, we removed 100 percent of the tumor and had no problems whatsoever."

I said, "Great. Thank you very much."

The doctor responded, saying, "Wait, wait. I don't think you understand what I'm telling you here. This was a challenging and delicate brain surgery. Normally, we don't have such positive feedback to share. But in your case, everything went perfectly. I think it's because we got in there so early," he continued. "Look, I know you had to push extremely hard to get this surgery, but what I'm telling you is if we didn't get in there to remove this tumor, which was holding and feeding the cancer, you would have had big problems. What I am telling you is that I think you may have just saved your own life!"

I think, dear reader, that there's an incredibly important lesson here, which is that sometimes, you really have to push hard for what you want or what you need. As others have told me, I hope that one, or hopefully many of you, dear readers, can apply this advice from this *old-school* construction worker in your own lives. He was a stranger to me, and he is a stranger to you. So what! Take his advice and use it in your own life right now, and I hope you will meet with great success just as I and others have done. As I write this, I feel a sense that God is telling me that my passing this on is going to be helpful to a lot of people who read this book—woo-hoo! I hope so!

Uncommon sense right now! Think about your life right now, especially areas where you feel frustrated, and ask yourself: What do you truly want or need? And once you decide what it is that you truly want or need, then resolve to go out into the world and push/push/push until you get what you want, and don't take "no" for an answer! Obviously, this advice doesn't work if what you're pushing for is stupid or unreasonable. As one of the chapters in this book highlights "how not to be a moron." If what you seek is reasonable and moral, then I believe you will likely find this advice to be a high-quality gift from God to you! Also, get yourself onto the "Right Now" Committee! That means don't delay anything. Attack this task with positive enthusiasm right now! Do it now!

CHAPTER 6

Intense Similarities Between 1775 and 2025

ASIDE FROM EVERYTHING THAT WAS GOING ON with me personally as I was first learning that I had brain cancer, I was—and still am—really struck by how much our current age—2024—is so incredibly similar to the time when Thomas Paine published his book *Common Sense*, in 1776. Similarly, as mentioned previously, both authors overcame life-threatening illnesses. Also, even though they are separated by 248 years, perhaps the intense *disunity* of our mutual life-threatening illnesses is, in a way, why and how we were/are both able to see commensurate disunity within the body politic.

As the author of *Uncommon Sense* in 2024, I see a vast commonality between 1775 and 2024, and that is just how dramatically bifurcated each era was in 1775 and now in 2024. In 1775, you were either a Patriot, supporting the newly formed United States of America, or a Loyalist, supporting that age's version of the deep state, otherwise known as King George. Tensions ran high, and there was (and now is) a pervasive feeling that "something's not right, and that we are on the cusp of profound and far-reaching change." In 2024, the bifurcation, more or less, is that you are either MAGA or Far Left, and, again, tensions are high, and there's a pervasive feeling, even explicitly called out in the media, that "something's not right and that we are all on the cusp of major change." It's astonishing how

15

similar these two time periods are, and I bet some intelligent and talented historians could probably present us with many more examples of the intense similarities between 1775 and 2024.

CHAPTER 7

"Maybe" and "I Don't Know" Are not Acceptable Answers

IN THIS NEXT CHAPTER, AND THROUGHOUT THIS book, I see value in highlighting the *old-school* advice from the blunt-speaking men I grew up with as a young boy in the 1970s. I have found over the years that all of this *old-school* advice is more relevant today than ever before, even in today's world, so I'd like to share some of it.

As this chapter title suggests, an important piece of advice I grew up with was my *old-school* male elders telling me "Maybe" and "I don't know" are not acceptable answers to any question, at any time. They would tell me: "I want an answer, not a fumble." Quite simply, I was never allowed to say "Maybe" or "I don't know."

And, again, due to the circumstances that I had brain cancer, in this next phase of the book, I found that, after the brain surgery, as I spoke to nurses and doctors and asked questions, I sometimes got weak answers. Frankly, I felt like I was getting a lot of "Maybes" and "I don't know's," and because I was literally facing life and death, I wasn't willing to accept these as credible answers. I continuously discerned that I would seek out new people or new resources to get my answers.

Here's what happened. Each and every day, I would go to the hospital for radiation therapy. While I was lying on the flat radiology table, the radiology technicians would attempt to kill the cancer cells by aiming and shooting their radiation gun. As they did this, I decided to meditate. After meditating, I felt as though I could sense or feel, or maybe, again, it was God speaking to me. Through this meditation, I felt that the cancerous cells inside my body were performing "evasive maneuvers" to "run away" from the radiation gun that was trying to kill them! Now of course, I didn't know this per se; it was just my brain thinking that anything under the threat of being killed would try to run away. If this was logical, I discerned, then wouldn't it be logical to assume that my cancerous cells would try to run away from the radiation gun that was trying to kill them? I thought this was an interesting thesis, and I wanted to discuss it with the radiologist and others, but each time I brought it up, she would just say, "Maybe" or "I don't know." I would calmly explain to her that this wasn't answering my questions.

I asked, "If these cancer cells, let's say, did try to run away from the radiation gun, is there a medication that you can give to me that would make the cancer cells "lethargic" so they couldn't run away? "Could they give me a medication that would essentially paralyze the cancer cells?" I'd ask. But I kept getting "Maybe" and "I don't know."

I started sharing my thesis with as many other people as I could find, and I was incredibly fortunate that my brother is a clinical research professor. As I shared these thoughts with him, he shared them with other researchers and started conducting research on his own. Lo and behold, he found some solid answers! He identified several medications, ancient Chinese and Indian herbs, supplements, and alternative therapies that would fulfill the goals I originated from meditating on the radiation table. Through this independent research, we identified numerous other recommendations to significantly improve the efficacy of both radiation and chemotherapy. What's more, he didn't just produce recommendations; he obtained solid clinical data that supported all his research, and all told, over the next few months, he made about twelve different recommendations to the neurologists, all with supporting clinical data. His recommendations focused on using clinically proven ancient herbs, supplements, and alternative therapies. My neurosurgical team accepted every recommendation we made, confirming the old-school advice that I learned as a child, which is that the words "Maybe" and "I don't know" are not acceptable answers—ever!

Dear reader, whenever you hear "Maybe" or "I don't know," take that as a signal from God, as I did, that you have to find someone else who will give you a real answer and not a fumble! One explicit example and recommendation found that if you increase the dosage and take a very commonly prescribed diabetes medication just prior to undergoing chemotherapy, the results would be that the chemotherapy would be significantly more effective. We made the recommendation, it was accepted, we implemented it, and then shortly after undergoing chemotherapy, my neurologist came to me, surprised but extremely positive. He said, "David, the chemotherapy is working better for you than we have ever seen it perform, and we're not really sure why. We've never seen it work this well! All we can say is that it must be because of the recommendation you and your brother made." This chief of neurology also told me that our work to try to make the cancer cells lethargic or paralyzed in the face of radiation was one of the latest clinical research techniques, which makes me think of additional *uncommon sense* advice I want to share with you below.

Dear reader: When this advice—or what I call "uncommon sense"—came into my brain, I felt it came from God just after this doctor spoke to me (and I share the advice below).

This neurologist went on to point out that they had accepted all our recommendations, and he felt everything we were doing had to be a big part of the reason why I was recovering so well. He said to me, "And you're giving us clinical data! We rarely get clinical data. We have a hard time obtaining clinical data, yet we're getting clinical data for every recommendation you make! How are you getting all this clinical data?" Here's what my tactic was: I told the chief of neurosurgery that what we tell the researchers is that we are working with one of the best and most respected cancer hospitals in the world, and if you make a recommendation, and the doctors accept it, they will give you credit for it. However, they require clinical data to even look at a recommendation, so if you don't provide us with clinical data, we can't even present it. With this approach and my brother's excellent work, we obtained lots and lots of clinical data. Now as I did in the preceding chapter, at the end of this section, I will provide some "uncommon sense" to benefit our dear readers; however, first, I have a jocular and funny aside.

One day, the chief of neurosurgery approached me in the hallway and said, "David, we recently gave you the maximum rates of radiation. That was hard to handle, but you handled it all very well. And then we prescribed for you the highest dosage of chemotherapy we've ever given and, again, that was very hard for you to handle, but you handled it all very well, so you're doing everything we ask of you. Thank you, and good job. But is there anything we can do for you?"

I said, "Yeah, how about some better-looking nurses?" Now for the first but not the last time, this chief of neurosurgery, a serious man, burst out into a great big laugh, and we both stood there having a great laugh!

He said, "See! See! That's it, David! This is why you're doing so well! It's because you have a great attitude," and he continued, "David, I'm serious. I'm not kidding you. I've seen too many patients do badly because they were not positive."

So, dear reader, before we go any further, please let me share the key lessons and advice from this section.

Uncommon sense advice number 1: One giant piece of advice that this story proves is about how, sometimes, a great idea—for example, trying to make my cancerous cells "lethargic" or paralyzed from running away from the radiation gun—can be worth its weight in gold. But how do you find this idea? I have found, with this experience as well as with many other examples throughout my thirty-five-year corporate career, sometimes, if not most times, the best advice is to realize that you, no matter who you are—and not a supposed "expert"—have the capability to originate the best idea. I have found, too, that whenever I quiet my mind and meditate, I frequently get great ideas. And importantly, as soon as the idea is shared, don't be surprised when you almost immediately hear people voice negativity. This is when you hear people tell you, "That won't work," or they'll say, "I've never heard that before!"

I feel like God was telling me, just like when hearing "Maybe" and "I don't know," that there should be red flags for you to find other people who will give you better answers. The key advice here is that whenever you hear people voicing negativity to you, that should be a red flag to get the opinions of others because we live in a world of far too much negative thinking, and you need to be on guard not to let it poison you!

In my example, I had a compelling idea that if we could paralyze the cancerous cells from "running away" from the radiation gun, that would be a great thing to do, and, thankfully, I didn't listen to all the morons telling me, "That won't work" or "I don't know," and then, someone found it compelling enough to research it. We ended up identifying, as my neurologist said, some of the best clinical research recommendations he's received in a very long time. So more uncommon sense: Be positive always, even if you have to force it. I mean, you know negativity isn't going to help you, ever, so just be positive. You don't even have to think about it.

Uncommon sense advice number 2: Don't be a baby. So I made a joke about wanting to see better-looking nurses. It was lighthearted and fun and didn't hurt a soul, so there's no problem. I say this because I shared this story with a good female friend. She told me I was out of line, and I explained it was a joke and that the doctor and I just had a good laugh, but she was adamant that I was being fresh, and she stopped speaking to me. That was almost a year ago. How incredibly stupid. So don't be a baby ass. Oh gee! Well, now, dear reader, please let me tell you one more funny aside. This was another time; through a little humor, I got my doctors to have a really big belly laugh!

One day, a doctor said to me, "Hey, David, we stopped giving you this medication. You don't have to take it anymore. We were giving it to you to help you avoid feeling confused, but I mean, really, are you confused?"

I said, "Yeah. I'm just confused why more really hot-looking women aren't just telling me they love me! Hahaha."

That was a good one, and my doctor had a good laugh, and then he got serious again and said something like, "Well, hmm, based upon your answer, I don't think we have any problems with you at all!" I took this all as a good sign from God. Hey, certainly, laughter is the best medicine!

Uncommon sense advice number 3: If your question is fair and important, don't accept "Maybe" and "I don't know" as answers at any time. Believe in yourself and find new people who will give you a credible answer. My experience is that the more you "reasonably push" for credible answers, the more you will find them, and the easier it will become. The more you will identify real, definitive benefits directly linked to you simply not accepting "Maybe" and "I don't know." Don't accept bullshit answers in life. Speak to other people, and you will find good, solid answers, and you will meet better people!

CHAPTER 8

Amnesia Wipeout: Meeting Yourself for the First Time

THIS WAS ONE OF THE DEFINING EXPERIENCES that gives me such a unique perspective today, as well as endowing me with a unique ability to address the complex and pressing issues of our times in the following chapters. Here, here's what happened next:

At this point in my brain cancer recovery, I had already pushed and received the exceptionally successful brain surgery that removed 100 percent of the cancerous tumor, and then I completed the ten weeks of radiation therapy. At this stage, I was working through eight weeks of chemotherapy. I was entering the hospital quite a bit, day after day. When you entered the hospital, the front desk clerk would ask, "What's your name? What's your birthday?" You were supposed to answer their questions, they would check you in on their computer, and they'd let you in. Simple enough. However, one day when they asked me, "What's your name? What's your birthday?" I froze. I couldn't remember.

I recall thinking it was really kind of absurd how I couldn't remember my own name. So I said to the hospital staff, "I'm sorry, but I'm having trouble remembering. Let me sit down for a minute."

The lady at the desk said, "Sure, no problem." I sat down for a good fifteen to twenty minutes and concentrated as hard as I could. I simply could not recall my own name. I had no idea when my birthday was—it seemed like such a hard question!

But then I felt a little panicked because I couldn't just remember my name; I didn't know who I was at all. I couldn't remember who my parents were, or where I went to school. I didn't know anything about myself! I remember putting my hand out in front of my face as if to prove to myself, "Okay, well, I'm here. I'm a person! Look, I can move my fingers." But I couldn't, for the life of me, recall what my name was or who I was. I didn't know anything about myself, so I stood up, walked over to the front desk, and told the lady, "I'm sorry, but I can't remember my name or my birthday.

The woman at the desk said, "That's okay. Let me ask you, do you have your wallet on you?" I searched my jacket's pockets, found my wallet, and said, "Yes, here it is."

She said, "Well then, let me ask, do you have a driver's license in your wallet?"

And I thought, "Ooh, now that's a good idea!" I fished around, found my license, and handed it to her.

She looked at it and said, "Okay, here's your name: You are David Albert Francoeur. Hello, David. It's nice to meet you." And then she told me to sit down while she called someone to come get me.

As I sat down, I felt there was something in the way she said, "Hello, David." It was like her voice just hung in the air, and it occurred to me that when she said, "Hello, David," her tone sounded very much like what you would expect the first time you met someone. But then, because I was experiencing a complete amnesia wipe out, I realized that this was the very first time I had ever heard my own name! I felt like this was the first time I ever met me! Now all I knew about myself was that my name was David, and that's because this front desk clerk just told me that's my first name.

From there, I remember going to the medical records office as I was trying to get my records. This meeting was difficult and bureaucratic, but I managed as best I could. After this meeting, I thought about the meeting, and more so about how I behaved during it. It was as if I was observing myself for the very first time. I was just learning about what kind of person I was because I was observing myself as someone entirely brand new, a complete stranger that I had literally just been introduced to for the very first time. So what I am telling you, dear reader, is that my brain was completely erased. I was a total stranger to myself, although I had the same physical body. From this point forward, I went through what I later realized to be a real gift from God, where, as an adult, I got introduced to myself, and for the very first time, and through a process of observation, I eventually learned who I am. But it was just an exceptionally weird, difficult, and rewarding process to essentially be rebooted. I remember, at this time, I was able to think and realize that, "Wow, this is really a serious and major deficit that I just absorbed, that I was overcome by a complete amnesia wipeout and that I had no memory whatsoever."

CHAPTER 9

My Dysfunction Hands Me a Massive Dividend!

FORTUNATELY, AT THIS TIME IN MY LIFE, and, as I will explain, I was a child of the 1970s. When I was growing up, all I heard was, "Boys don't cry" and "Boys don't show their emotions." So I didn't! But as I grew up, and only after this time with my brain cancer, I think some kind of switch turned on in my body, soul, and spirit. What I mean is, as I grew up, I don't think I ever really, or even minimally, felt my emotions at all. I could think, but I really didn't feel. I remember once being in a philosophy class in college when the professor asked all of us, "What do you feel?" I kept telling him what I thought. Finally, the professor said to me, "No, David. You keep telling me what you think, but I'm asking you, what do you feel?"

I remember thinking, "What the hell is he talking about?" I stopped and tried to connect with my feelings, but then, I turned to him and said, "I don't feel anything." But the truth was, while I guess I must have had emotions, I never, ever felt my emotions, and this is where this dysfunction yielded me a gigantic *peace dividend*, so to speak. I'll tell you what this peace dividend was, but then I need to tell you that, right around this time, it felt like someone flipped a switch, and suddenly, I started feeling my emotions. But first, the peace dividend!

So as I was speaking to the hospital front desk clerk, she was extremely nice to me, and I think very sensitively to the fact that here I was, someone who didn't know his own name and who couldn't answer any basic questions about who he was, where he lived, who were his parents, etc. The peace dividend was a direct benefit to me—dysfunctionally, not being able to feel my emotions because, at this moment where the front desk clerk revealed to me the enormity of the fact that I was suffering from complete amnesia. As I couldn't feel, I thought, "Hey, David. Just take this big problem and flip it on its head. It's not a problem! It's a giant benefit! Think of it that way." I quickly convinced myself. I remember sitting by myself in the hospital lobby chair, grappling with all of this, and I thought, "This is fantastic! This is a giant gift from God! You get to learn who you are as if you are a complete stranger to yourself, and, hey, why not just think that this is, actually, really pretty cool!" So from then on, I carried on and, contrary to not feeling badly in any way, I felt joy; at least, I thought joyfully. I "felt" like I was fortunate that God was giving me this terrific gift!

Several weeks down the road, after returning to the rehabilitation center, I experienced feeling my emotions daily, really for the first time in my life. But for now, I can look back and say I truly benefitted from the "Boys don't cry" dysfunctional upbringing I had, and, hey, that's okay! I am very grateful that this dysfunction was able to assist me in this way. The bottom line is once I realized that I was undergoing complete amnesia, I didn't feel upset or badly at all. On the contrary, and I think dysfunctionally, I felt lucky and very fortunate!

Uncommon sense: If you concentrate, dear reader, can you put yourself in a position where you are observing yourself today for the very first time? What would you observe about yourself? What would you say are some very good traits you have in your behaviors? And likewise, what would be some areas where you could use improvement? My story is just a story from someone you don't even know, but I think anyone can benefit from my experience. Think about your own behavior at any given moment and then ask yourself what you would notice about yourself if you were meeting yourself for the very first time? Just try it. Also, my experience demonstrates the extreme helpfulness and power of stoic philosophy, which states that while you cannot control what happens to you, you can very much control how you react to it!

Dear reader: We're now at a point in this book where I feel like I've explained to you my early experiences, my first experiences where I was told by a sophisticated medical community that I was going to die, and then how I had to push/push/push to get lifesaving brain surgery, and also how I twisted the amnesia wipeout from something bad into something highly beneficial.

CHAPTER 10

Male Emotions: Is This a Chemical Imbalance?

AT THIS POINT IN MY STORY, I was living at a rehabilitation center, and I was feeling better, especially because my memory was beginning to come back to me. I was feeling like myself again. Then I noticed when I woke up in the morning, something was different, and I really couldn't quite put my finger on it. As I had been experiencing, I felt God telling me something, and what he told me was that "He had opened the window." I kept hearing this over and over for days or a couple of weeks. Then one day, I spoke to one of the therapists at the rehab center, and, in responding to all his questions and by just trying to tell him what I was experiencing, he said to me, "David, it just sounds like you're feeling your feelings," and again, I had no idea what that meant.

I am a smart guy. I went to college, and I've held numerous executive-level jobs. In 1998, I was the youngest in the nation to run for U.S. Congress, but even to hear the word *feelings*, I really didn't know what feelings were. Soon, each day, when I woke up, I felt feelings for the first time in my life.

In the beginning, I enjoyed it because I felt happy feelings, but then, at one point, I started to feel some negative emotions, like sadness or hurt. I remember thinking: "I don't like this at all," but as I tried to transition back to just thinking, I thought: "Somehow, we let the genie out of the bottle, but I want to put the genie back into the bottle." I thought I could fix it! So one day, I connected with one of the doctors. I asked the doctor, "What are feelings?" He tried to give me an answer, but I couldn't fathom what feelings were, again, because I don't think I ever truly felt my feelings. I kept asking questions, trying to narrow it down to something I could understand. I remember asking, "Is it a chemical imbalance?" and "How do we fix this?" Each day became a wild emotional roller-coaster ride for me. I was feeling all my emotions, and truth be told, I determined two things.

First, even though I found emotions either unpleasant or unnecessary, I also started feeling more connected and more *present* in life. I felt, okay, this is good, but after a few weeks, I had had enough. Fortunately, one day, as I was in the cafeteria having a coffee, I started speaking with a ninety-four-year-old gentleman. He asked me what was going on with me, and we spoke all morning and most of the afternoon. By late afternoon, I said to him, "Okay, so can you give me some advice?"

He said, "I think, as a man, you can simply decide to switch off your emotions, so if you want to turn them off, just turn them off!" As I write this, it sounds vague, but at the time, I knew exactly what he meant.

Later that night, I was in my bedroom lying in bed, and I thought, "Okay, that's it. I'm turning off all my emotions right now." Bam! Done! And that was that, so long as I consciously knew I turned off my emotions, I really didn't feel my emotions. But then I got greedy and thought, "Well, I'd like to feel the good emotions but not the bad emotions, and I tried to make this happen, but I couldn't."

I found out then, and I am still this way today; if I want to, I can pretty much shut off all my emotions, but I can't pick and choose individual emotions. It's either all or nothing. Honestly, it felt great to turn them all off and not have to deal with them. Now it's hard for me to truly know 100 percent, but I can still turn off all my emotions if I want to; at the same time, I generally feel a lot of my emotions. I have learned how to live not just with my emotions but to live well, and this feels so weird to say, but actually to value my feelings. Every once in a while, I take a "vacation" and turn them all off, but I haven't done this in a long time, so maybe now I am just okay?

I have both spoken to and observed a lot of my male friends who struggle with emotions just as I did. Just as I could never understand someone who told me they're a highly emotional person, I know a lot of people may have trouble understanding the serious damage of raising boys, telling them constantly that they shouldn't feel or express their feelings, and then get surprised by how challenged many men are with all this. I feel compelled to say that, as I observe the world of 2024, it just really seems like men are not, in general, permitted to share their feelings. I experience myself with a great many people, but particularly women, that I am simply shamed if I ever share my feelings.

Uncommon sense: My thinking here is that, generally speaking, nice people, kind people, and people who are not morons will well be able to handle themselves and others emotionally well. It's always the same thing: it's just the unkind, uncaring, and difficult people who cause trouble. The only way I truly discern how to deal with this is to disengage and avoid unkind, uncaring, and difficult people! That sounds simple enough, but as I was grappling with emotions, one therapist told me, "David, as I speak to you, I can see that you have never invested any energy into protecting your emotional health!" Wow. He was completely correct, and once he brought this to my attention, I really started to value my emotional well-being, something I had never done before, and this, mostly, took the form of me cutting the toxic people out of my life. I want to say something to anyone reading this: if you have toxic people in your life, my experience is that, while it can be very difficult to disengage, it's worth it. Life isn't meant to be wasted on toxic people, and I sincerely wish anyone who wants to walk down their own road to better protect their emotional well-being, do so. Good luck and Godspeed! You will find better outcomes. Have faith, and fix it!

CHAPTER 11

Politically Incorrect Advice on Gender Relations

At this point, I was out of the hospital and staying at a rehabilitation center, which was more of a nursing home for recovering patients. At the rehab center, there were a lot of patients in their nineties, and, as I am a social person, I soon found myself making a lot of friends and speaking for long periods of time with many very nice people who were ninety-one, ninety-three, ninety-four, and older. It was a wonderful experience.

As I "reentered the world," my first experience was unusual in that I started receiving the same politically incorrect advice from a wide assortment of many different people who didn't even know each other, both male and female. I'll tell you the advice right now, and I think you will be just as shocked by it as I was the first time I heard it. I was shocked, and at first, I thought it was just plain stupid. But, as time passed, I kept encountering one problem after another, as so many people told me I would. Eventually, I started to implement the advice, and unfortunately, I found this stupid and politically incorrect advice to work surprisingly well.

Okay, you've waited long enough, so here's the advice I was receiving at this point in my brain cancer recovery. I feel hesitant to give it to you because I feel like I will be erroneously criticized for being sexist. I am not. I have a lot of female friends, and I have worked with a lot of smart, competent, and nice women. So let's do this: Just take the advice at face value, and as you go about your life, as I did, experiment with it. Like everything else in this world, you may find that it helps you a lot, or you may find it doesn't apply to you at all. So what! Just hear it, and do whatever you want!

The advice was this: "If you want a good life, a life free of trouble and difficulty and grief, you just have to accept the fact that you have to stop speaking to and interacting with all women!" Whoa! I know it sounds crazy! I can't say that I always follow this advice, but selectively, at times, I do. I am judicious about how much I follow it and, for me, I have decided to just be more observant. For example, if I stop following this advice altogether but then find I keep running into one problem after another, I start to follow it again. So I just toggle it on and off, and I'm hoping this issue will disappear!

Just after receiving this politically incorrect advice from a medical professional from either the hospital or the rehabilitation center, a few days later, while I had all this in my mind, I went to the bank to cash a check. So I walked into my bank and walked up to one of the tellers. As soon as I got there, I noticed that there were also male bank tellers who were available, but I had quickly walked up to the closest teller, who was female. I remember I thought about the advice to not interact with any woman, but I decided "the heck with it," and I started conversing with the female teller. I said, "Hi, I'm a customer here, and I have this check for $3,500. I'd like to cash it and deposit $2,000 into my existing checking account, and then I'd like the remaining $1,500 back in cash in $50 bills."

She took the check and, after a few minutes, she, somewhat tersely, handed it back to me and just said, "I can't."

I asked, "You can't? Why not?" And she said, "I can't cash the check."

I asked, "Why can't you cash the check?" Again, she just said impolitely, "I can't cash the check."

I said, "I hear you saying you can't cash the check, but what I'm asking you is, 'Why? Why can't you cash the check?'"

And, for the last time, full of consternation, she said, "I said, 'I can't!'"

So I said, "Okay, look, I'm a customer of this bank. I have a bank account here, and I have this check that I want to cash, so here, please cash my check." Then she goes utterly mute and stops interacting with me whatsoever.

I very politely responded, "Let me ask you something else. Is there a man here I can talk to?"

Madly, she quipped, "What do you mean a *man*?"

I said, "Well, you tell me that you can't help me, so I'm just wondering if there's a male teller here that I can speak to?"

She agitatedly said, "Do you really think that speaking to a man will solve all your problems?"

And being frustrated with this whole experience, I answered calmly but with brutal honesty by saying, "Yes, I do think that if I speak to a man, he will eliminate any problems."

She instantly started speaking harshly to me, so the last thing I said was, "I don't believe I have a banking problem."

"What do you mean?" she asked.

I said, "I don't believe I have any banking problems." I knew I was out on a limb, but I said, "I don't have any banking problems that stop you from cashing the check. The only problem I have," I continued, "is that I am speaking with a woman." I realized then and now that this was too forward for me to say; however, I was legitimately frustrated by her gross incompetence and consistently bad attitude. Unsurprisingly, she became instantly extremely upset, and she began to cuss me out. She was speaking loudly, and we were both standing in a bank lobby covered in granite, with high ceilings, so the acoustics were such that her voice was significantly amplified. Because she was speaking so harshly, it all sounded loud and horrible.

Standing there, I thought, "All I want to do is to cash a check. How can it be this big of a problem?" But because she was so loud and so rude, I noticed that quite a few other bank customers were looking at us.

In short, this female teller was causing a scene, and right then, I thought, "Well, there's probably no better way to speak to a manager than to just let this woman continue to act so badly that, at some point, a manager will come out."

And sure enough, within a minute or two, which seemed like an eternity, a man in a suit came walking toward us very quickly while saying, "What is going on here? What is going on here?"

"Thank God, it's the manager," I thought as he walked right up to the teller and me.

He looked at the teller and asked, "What is going on here? Why are you speaking to this person this way?"

The teller looked directly at him and said absolutely nothing.

Again, he asked, "Excuse me. I asked you a question. Why are you speaking to this man this way?" And, once again, she said nothing. So finally, the manager turned to me and said, "Excuse me, sir. I'm sorry to bother you with this, but do you mind telling me what's going on here?"

I responded, "Sure. I asked her to cash my check, deposit $2,000 into my existing account, and give me the rest back in all $50s. She said she can't. I asked her several times why she couldn't cash my check, but she wouldn't answer me. So I asked if I could speak to a male teller, and with that, she got upset and started speaking to me this way, and that's where we are."

The manager replied, "Okay, thanks. Do you have the check on you?"

I said, "Yes."

"Can I see it?" the manager asked, and I immediately handed him the check. He responded, "Give me a minute," and stepped behind the counter. A few minutes later, he returned and said, "David, here's the situation. The person who wrote you this check has a restriction on his account. All that means is that before I can cash the check, I have to call him to get his verbal permission to cash it. Do I have your permission to call him?"

"Sure, no problem," I immediately responded. The manager immediately called and asked if he could cash the check, to which the checkwriter immediately approved. He hung up the phone, turned to me, and said, "Please give me one more minute." A minute later, he said, "Here you go, David. Here's your receipt for the $2,000 deposited into your existing checking account, and here's the remaining $1,500 in all $50s. I think we're all done here now, right?"

I said, "Yes, and thank you. Thank you very much." At this point, the female teller—I'm not kidding—rebutted, "See, I told you speaking to a man wasn't going to help you!" I am done relaying this story to you; take from it what you will.

Related to all talk about the genders is a relatively new trend, wildly discriminatory, and that is the incredibly strong anti-male hysteria gripping our society right now. It is so far overblown that I read in the media that our society has the lowest marriage rates on record and the lowest birth rates on record. I saw an online poll saying that over 80 percent of single men would rather be alone than have to deal with all of the trouble of dating women. This is a crisis situation, and it's plain for all to see. It's cancel culture run amok. But my observation, as a student of history, is that I believe we live in a fairly self-correcting society. As is commonly said, the anti-male pendulum has now swung so far in one direction; as sure as the sun will rise tomorrow, I believe the pendulum will soon self-correct. I think this is something akin to the natural rhythm in both the physical and social worlds.

Here's another story on gender relations. At this point, *I was staying in the hospital, and they had situated my hospital bed close to the hallway door. I could overhear a lot of people in the hallway having a boisterous conversation. I kept hearing people talk about a "GN score,"* so I opened the door and asked the male nurse, "What is a 'GN score'?"

And he said, "Well, I'll tell you, but please keep it confidential. The GN Score stands for the General Nonsense Index."

I said, "I'm sorry, but I'm not following. What are you saying?"

He responded, "We work in this large hospital, right? And there are a lot of female employees. But, unfortunately, we find that many of the women who work here don't do their jobs or don't do them well. They often cause problems for the patients, sometimes even serious problems. Dear reader, please let me interject here to say that my nurses who work in the neurology department all excellent, exceptionally competent, caring, and helpful!

"As a guy, I find that many times, these problems are later blamed on the men, so we get in trouble for the fact that so many women don't do their jobs. We created a rating system used to rate

36

all the women we work with. It's called the General Nonsense Index. We use this rating scale to rate every single woman we come in contact with, and if she scores higher than 90 points, all of the men who work with her stop all contact with this person. We won't work with her or speak with her at all. It's the only way we've been able to figure out how to work with women."

Surprised to hear this, but more curious to understand how the GN Index works, I replied, "Wow! How does it work?"

He said, "There are three questions that you ask, and for each question, you rate the woman by giving her from 0 to 35 points depending on how much she either adheres to the question or not. So if she isn't at all what the question is asking, you give her 0 points. If she is very much behaving as the question asks, you give her up to 35 points. At the end of asking these three questions, you add up all the points, and if she scores over 90, then our experience is she's just too difficult and not worth working with. Therefore, you should just completely stop all interaction with her."

He replied, "Funny thing is, I've shared this system with many people. Now that you know it, you'll find yourself using it with every woman in your life. We know from much experience and discussion that the scoring system works exceptionally well. We have never met a woman who scores over 90 points with whom you can effectively interact, so try it," he said.

I asked, "What are the three questions that you ask?"

He responded, "Okay, the first question is this: Is she illogical?" Then he quickly added, "You shouldn't have to think a lot about this when you run through these questions here. With this question, we mean, I'm sure you've met some women who, when they're speaking, you're thinking, "OMG, what they're saying is just plain illogical!" That's what we mean here. If they're really, frequently illogical, you can give her up to 35 points. Give her between 0 and 35 points depending on how illogical you think she is.

"The next question is this: Is she nonsensical? In this case, you might think she's not illogical, but what she says doesn't make much sense. It's nonsensical. It's the same thing; give her from 0 to 35 points based on how nonsensical she is. Then the last question. This last question is the only question where you can break the rating scale. With this question, you can assign as many as 100 points, so instead of assigning between 0 and 35 points, with this third question, you can assign from 0 to 100 points. So a woman can be logical and sensical. However, if she rates badly enough in this third question, she can still tip her total score to over 90 points, which calls for you to completely eliminate all interaction with her moving forward."

"Okay," I said. "You've piqued my interest! What's the third question?"

He replied, "The third question is: Is she just plain difficult?" He then explained, "What we mean here is there are just too many women who get too upset too often, where everything's a problem, and/or they're just so incompetent that they can't do anything right. That's what we mean by just being difficult. So there you have it. That's the GN Score Index."

Dear reader, I had many more experiences at the hospital. Finally, I was discharged back to the rehabilitation center for a few weeks.

The day I got back to the rehab center, I walked into my bedroom and found another roommate, this time a younger man of about forty years old. Surprisingly, he immediately told me something very similar. He said, "This is a place where none of the women do their jobs, but all of the men are very helpful." He mentioned, "It can get difficult to manage, but I've invented a game called "the Gameshow,' which at least gives us something interesting to do."

"Okay, how do you play this game?" I asked.

He replied, "Well, let's say you want something, so you ask one of the nurses. But if you ask a female nurse, chances are she will immediately start her response to you by saying 'Unfortunately,' and then she will tell you why she can't do what you ask. Seriously, I've been here for a long time, and this is all they do." He explained, "But that begins 'the Gameshow!'" When he said the word *Gameshow*, he sang a little jingle as if we were watching this on TV. He was making this fun and funny! He continued, "We play 'the Gameshow' by going into the hallway and getting a male nurse or a male orderly. Get any male, even if he's the janitor. You just need to get any male and ask him to come into the room. When the male walks into the room, you ask him the same exact question that you just asked the female nurse, using exactly the same words, and then we watch what happens."

I said, "Okay, but I'm curious. You say you've played this game a lot. What usually happens?"

My rehab center roommate responded, "Well, most, if not all, of the females, will tell you how they can't do what you're asking or they'll say nothing and just leave, and most, if not all, of the men, will do the exact opposite. They will all say something like, 'Yes, sir. Let me get that for you right now.'"

I thought it would be good if, at some point, we could actually come up with some prizes to give out to the participants of this game, but we probably can't do that. I don't know why, but I find it fun and interesting to play this game I call "the Gameshow!"

Dear reader, I'll make this brief, but here's how this section ends:

At one point during my stay at the rehabilitation center, they kept having a lot of problems with their kitchen. I never learned exactly what the problems were, but for long periods of time, they didn't serve any food: no breakfast, no lunch, no dinner, and no snacks! One day, for twenty-four hours, I didn't get a shred of food, absolutely nothing. When the next day rolled around, we had reached more than a period of thirty-six hours—a day and a half—where I hadn't had any food whatsoever. I was just exceptionally hungry. A female nurse walked into my bedroom, and I said to her, "Excuse me, but I know you have a problem with the kitchen, but I haven't received any food all day yesterday and so far today. We're at about thirty-six hours where I haven't eaten a thing, and I'm just crazy hungry!" I started to say, "So what I wanted to ask is..." but the female nurse wouldn't let me finish speaking.

She interrupted by saying, "Unfortunately ..." and with her saying this one first word, my roommate sang out, "And the Gameshow begins! Da-da-da-da-daaa!"

The nurse looked at him, wondering what he was talking about. My roommate said to the female, "Okay, thanks. We're all set. Never mind."

But, in the spirit of the game, I said, "Wait, first let me ask her…" And I said to the female nurse, "I know that you have kitchen problems, but I was told that if I was really hungry, you could just go down to the kitchen and ask them if they can make me a ham and cheese sandwich. I was told that the kitchen will always try to give you a sandwich, even if they're not serving food."

But, again, almost instantly, the female nurse told me, "No." She couldn't do that. There was nothing she could do, and I'd have to go without food. My roommate said he'd like to speak to me alone and asked her to leave, which she did.

I went to the hallway but came back into my bedroom and told my roommate that I didn't see any male nurses in the hallway, so there was no one I could ask.

My roommate was a real joker, and he started singing that it was now "a special edition of the Gameshow," and he sang little jingles. He then turned to me and said, "Okay, now we're really going to test out our gender analysis here!" He said, "Go into the hallway and find any man. I don't care if he's not a nurse. Go get the janitor. Get any man!"

I returned to the hallway, which was loaded with female nurses. I located one guy with an orange vest mopping the floor. I approached him and said, "My roommate and I have a question and were just wondering if you could step into our room so we can ask you a question?"

He immediately responded, "Sure, no problem."

He followed me into the bedroom. As soon as we entered, my roommate yelled out and sang "And the Gameshow continues!"

I looked at this maintenance worker, and I explained my problem: that I hadn't eaten in thirty-six hours, and I was crazy hungry! I said, "I was told that if I was really hungry, you could just go down to the kitchen and ask them if they could make me a ham and cheese sandwich. I was told that the kitchen will always try to give you a sandwich, even if they're not serving food."

The maintenance man, who looked to be in his fifties, immediately said, "Sure, worth a try. I'll go ask them right now, and then I'll come back, okay?"

I said, "Yes, thank you."

The man left, and about twenty-five minutes later, he returned. He came into my bedroom and said, "I think you're going to be happy with what I was able to do!" He continued, "I went into the kitchen and told the kitchen staff that I had a patient who was really, really hungry and could they just give me a ham and cheese sandwich? And the kitchen guys said, 'Sure, do you want two sandwiches?' So I figured that you said you were really hungry, so I got you two sandwiches." He said, "I told the kitchen guys that I don't know what you want on your sandwich, but can they just set me up with something good?" He said, "So the kitchen guys gave you a couple of plastic bags filled with lettuce and onions and pickles. I got you a couple of small containers filled with mayo and mustard."

I started to thank him, but he cut me off and said, "Wait! Wait. Then as I was walking around the kitchen, I found a counter that had a large basket of small bags of potato chips, so I asked if I could take a bag of chips." The maintenance guy continued speaking, "The kitchen guys were really good. They said, 'Just help yourself to whatever you want!'" He said, "So I got you two ham and cheese sandwiches and two bags of chips, but then, I figured you need something to drink, and they told me to help myself, so I just kept walking around the kitchen, and I found some small bottles of Diet Coke. So I got you two small plastic bottles of Diet Coke, and I found some ice, so here's a big glass of ice too! That's it, huh? So how'd I do?"

I remember saying to this guy, and I truly meant it, "Hey, man, I can't thank you enough. To say you did excellent isn't good enough. I mean, two sandwiches, two bags of chips, and Diet Coke! I'm amazed! I'm so hungry, and you have helped me out so much. Thank you very much!"

He said, "It was my pleasure, and I'm working here for another two to three hours, so if you want anything else, just come into the hallway to find me, and I'm happy to help you again!"

So this is the end of this section on gender relations. Still, my experiences, every week and almost every day, continue to make me really feel, or observe, that there is a major trend unfolding in our society today. It is one that is anti-male, but there is another aspect whereby, I don't know why, but the level of kindness, competence, or just plain responsibility of women is hitting the wall. I think this overall poor showing with so many women is a real problem where I already see negative repercussions unfolding in society, and these repercussions are hurting more than anyone else, women, not men. My belief is as trends unfold in our society, we usually see a trend unfold for at least a short time before it becomes presented across the media. But then, after a short time, it hits the media, and then we see it widely presented in the media, and finally, it's saturated in the media. For the first time ever, I have just started to see an article here or two calling out, primarily, poor female behavior. And then, beginning in the fourth quarter of 2023, I see almost weekly more and more articles specifically highlighting female bad behavior and so on. So what I am saying is that I believe there's a major sociological trend emerging across the major media and society. Like most things, I think this trend has some legitimate causes, and I also think it's hard to know what is really going on. So we'll just have to discuss as much as we can.

Here's how I would explain it: I think a very large part of the problem was that, not too long ago, feminism was completely rede-fined by feminists themselves. They told women repeatedly and aggressively that, in these modern times, women shouldn't look to just be good wives and mothers and to run a good household. No, they said that you should be able to have your kids and be a nice mother and wife and have all that. But you should also expect to have your career, so you stay being a career woman. And now what we find just by searching online, we find a lot of women of all ages and demographics saying this feminist outcome is just very unlikely, if not impossible to achieve. I find this whole issue so absurd because as a guy who speaks with many friends and other male acquaintances, I can honestly say that as I was one of those traditional married men who was the sole financial provider, I made all the money, did all the food shopping, cooking, and a large share of house cleaning, laundry, chores, and the traditional roles as previously defined—the man goes to work and provides a good solid infrastructure for his entire family. And the woman takes charge of running the household and caring and supporting her husband and her children. Today, this trend has it that women—rightly—cite the idea that they can "have it all" by being in charge of the household and by keeping full-time career. Well, most women and men today can see that this is an absurd idea. You can either work full-time or be in charge of running the household, but to actually try to do both is just a fool's game because it's really saying the omen will work "double full-time." So I think this stupid, "expert" advice has, in reality, destroyed a lot of husbands and wives' lives by just getting couples overextended in ways that don't lead to success.

CHAPTER 12

Race Relations: An Outrageously Positive Story

ALL IN ALL, I SPENT A GOOD four to six weeks living at a rehabilitation center, and this is where my "race relations" experience was revealed to me in a very forceful way! During my time living at the rehabilitation center, I frequently noticed that when I woke up in the morning, I would, in no uncertain terms, feel as though God was speaking directly to me. His voice would just come into my head, and he would always speak very clearly and matter-of-factly. It was just clear and unambiguous but never with any emotion. At first, the Voice told me, "David, I have many things I want to reveal to you, and if you will just listen and do your best to look, listen, and learn, you will become a better person." And then, on a daily basis, he started telling me things about the day ahead. He would always pick out people in my life; they could be family or strangers, but somehow, he would always tell me to either invest my energy in speaking with someone, or he would tell me specific people that I should steer clear of and stay away from any interaction.

His speech was always matter-of-fact, short, and direct. He would say things like, "You're going to have a good experience speaking with this person today," or, "Don't speak to this person. They will be nothing but trouble for you today." I began to notice that everything he told me came true. Everything unfolded precisely the way he would describe it! And then one morning, I woke up, and, I'm not kidding, the Voice of God came to me, and he said, "David, today I am going to send you a gift! It's something that you've wanted for a very long time, and you've been asking people to bring it to you, but nobody has. Today, I am going to send you this as a gift!"

As soon as I felt/heard this, I remember thinking, "Okay, that's it! This has to be my brain playing tricks on me because, come on, I can't believe God is telling me he's going to send me a gift!" It seemed too fantastical to be true. And then I remember, in the very instant that I thought this: God said to me, "You have to believe in me," and then, within thirty seconds, a nurse came into my room and said, "David, here you go," as she handed me a large Post Office delivery envelope.

I asked, "What is this?"

And she said, "The postman just came to deliver it, and it's addressed to you. That's all I know."

So I took the envelope and opened it. Inside was a very nicely packaged gift! I had been asking for someone to bring me a disposable razor for weeks so I could shave, but no one would bring me one, and I had a thick beard—I just really wanted to shave. As I opened the envelope, I was struck by how caringly the envelope was packed. The envelope included not just a nice disposable razor but also a travel-size can of shaving cream and a small bottle of after-shave lotion. Wow! It was precisely what I had been wanting and asking for for weeks, and it was all packaged up as a lovely gift! It was, in other words, precisely what God had just told me: he was going to deliver to me! Again, wow! It turned out, I later discovered, that it was sent to me by a friend I had recently spoken to, but I can't overlook that it seemed to be the work of God!

I shaved, and that felt great, but of course, I was still very, very upset about being erroneously told by a female hospital nurse, who just really got her facts wrong, that I would be dead within a few short weeks! Later that night, this is where my outrageously positive race relations story begins: I was alone in my rehabilitation bedroom, and I was upset. I think I probably looked like I was very upset.

As I mentioned previously, as a boy raised in the 1970s who was always told, "Boys don't cry," I still today feel a bit shy to tell you… I shed a tear! And as I sat alone in my bedroom and shed this tear, one of the young Black male nurses walked in and saw me! There were a lot of Black male nurses at this facility. This Black nurse walked in and took a good look at me. He looked me squarely in the eyes and then took a step back, pointed at me, and gave me a rousing, energetic, and very positive pep talk! He said, "Let me tell you something! You is good! You is strong, and you're going to beat whatever it is that you have!" And he kept going. He gave me an incredibly kind and caring, high-energy pep talk for a good twenty minutes! And that's not all! He returned to see me in my room every night for many days, and he always gave me a rousingly positive pep talk!

You can't see right now, dear reader, but I'm getting choked up just thinking about what I'm writing! As I said, I was just told I would be dead in a matter of weeks, and here was a guy who I didn't know at all, a complete stranger, and yet, he must have sensed I was a worried soul, and he treated me with such kindness and concern, more kindness and concern than I was getting from anybody else! I never even got his name, but I will never forget him, and I feel as though someday, in Heaven, we will shake hands and be friends!

Now here is a little something I noticed in our world today. I'm not quite sure what it means, but I feel there's some reason why it was revealed to me. As this nurse continued coming into my room each night, on many nights, there would also be a female nurse in my room. When the young, black, male nurse who was giving me the pep talk would leave, the female nurse would always ask, "Who was that?" I'd tell her, "I don't know, just one of the other nurses."

"Why is he coming in here and speaking with you?" the female nurse would ask.

And I would say, "Well, I think it's because he knows I'm having a tough time, so he's just being nice and helpful."

But the female nurse would always keep asking me questions, but in a way that was as if there was a problem. "Why is he coming here? How do you know him? Why is he being nice to you?"

Finally, I had to ask the female nurse just to leave. She seemed offended that I was frustrated with her questions, so I said, "This guy is just being nice to me. It's really an extraordinary act of kindness, so why do you keep asking me questions as if there's something wrong? Is there a problem?" After asking me so many questions, she appeared very offended that I asked her a question, and then she turned, left the room in a huff, and I never saw her again. The black male nurse came back the next night, and I had a chance to speak with him and thank him.

He said something back to me like, "Of course! This is how people are supposed to be, right?"

The following morning, I woke up, and God said to me, "David, I have something big to reveal to you today! You're going to like it."

So here's what this is all about. I'd been staying at this rehabilitation center for several weeks now, and this rehab center was just one very long hallway with bedrooms on each side and a cafeteria at the end of the hall. I found myself walking in the hallway quite a bit every day. But what I found is, again, with all the young Black male nurses, whenever I walked down the hallway, these young Black male nurses and I couldn't pass each other in the hallway without shaking hands, backslapping, or fist-bumping. Each and every single time— dozens of times per day—whenever a Black nurse and I saw each other, we'd immediately backslap, shake hands, fist-bump, and talk.

We never, not even once, missed doing this. Then one day, I was walking down the hall just after the head nurse told me I was going to be discharged. I was going to be able to go home! So as I walked down the hall, I must have had some kind of look on my face because one of the Black guys saw me and yelled out, "Yo, David, what's up, man? What are you doing?"

I responded, "Hey, man. They're discharging me. They told me I'm going home today!"

"What?" he yelled, and then he put his head up and looked all the way down the hallway and shouted, "Hey, everyone. It's David, man. He's leaving us!"

And from the far end of the hallway, I heard some guys yelling, "No!" A minute or so later, I looked down this very long hallway and, starting at the far end, I saw about fifteen Black male nurses all gathering in a bunch, and then they all started running down the hall toward me! I didn't understand what was happening and didn't know what to expect. These guys were all hooting and hollering as they ran straight toward me! As they ran up to me, we started backslapping, talking, shaking hands, smiling, laughing, and expressing great friendship and camaraderie. We were all telling each other how good the other guy was. It couldn't have been a friendlier gathering, full of outrageously intense camaraderie, goodwill, genuine friendship, and respect.

As I was being hugged and backslapped by so many, I couldn't help but notice that some of the guys were actually tearing up. We didn't want to say goodbye to each other, and we all felt a great sense of loss. It was both joyous and heartbreaking. It had become very emotional when several nurses and doctors came up and started pulling on my sleeves, trying to get me to walk out the door to be discharged. But the more they pulled on me to leave, the more these guys held onto me and wouldn't let me go! At one point, all of us, being, for lack of a better term, red-blooded men, felt like these guys and I were going to fight the doctors and nurses. I don't say this in a bad way at all; it's just with all the tussling, I think all of us felt like it'd be fun if we got in a punch-up. But of course, at one point, the guys let me go, and the doctors and nurses rather quickly pulled me away.

I'll never forget—I'm getting choked up again—I'll never forget looking at all their faces. We all felt genuine heartbreak! In that moment, and many times since then, I have reflected on this and thought, "Wow! On one of the toughest days of my life, I was surrounded not just by friends but by a large group of truly best friends." The irony is that all these great friends were really all strangers I had just met! Then I walked outside and told one of the male doctors, "Gee, you really know how to send a guy off!"

And he said, "David, that's never happened before. You have touched a lot of people! I can honestly say that this was one of the best experiences of my entire life." Not to spoil this, but as this experience was ending, several female nurses gathered around me, all with expressions of consternation, and they wanted to know, "Why were these guys acting this way?" "How do you know them?"

To which I exasperatingly said, "Does it really matter?"

That experience is something I will never forget. But I also think, as first revealed to me by God when I first woke up and now that I am fortunate enough, and well enough, to write this book. Please let me say what I think are some good lessons for the world in this story. And that is, we are all connected, and often, there is great, natural, organic friendship and mutual respect. It's not just the way things should be; it's the way things are! I think most people, the vast majority of people, want to and are well able to get along. Of course, there's more work to be done, but in some ways, there seems to be less of a problem among people than what we read in the media.

Why? I don't know. There is a problem with a minority of morons who, instead of supporting events like this, ask stupid questions like, "Why are you guys friends?"

I think, as I said, "God told me he wanted to reveal something big to me, and then, this is what he showed me." Now that you know the story of what was revealed, what do you think are the key learnings? What do you pull away from this story?

Uncommon sense: We are all God's children, and there is value in every single person. Racism is for stupid people who don't know any better. Everyone should be judged, as a truly great man once said, on the content of their character and not by the color of their skin, or for that matter, by their gender, or their sexual orientation, or anything—just on the content of their character! So true. This event also revealed to me that there is massive organic positive goodwill among a great many people. We need to figure out a way in our society to allow all this goodwill to come forward, just as the backslapping and goodwill naturally flowed forward in my relations with all the black male nurses at this rehab center! Thank you, God, for giving me this experience and allowing me to share it here in this book! It's an outrageously positive story on race relations. I hope we start to see a lot more positive news and results in the media too.

Dear reader, that's my section on race relations. I have one last story to share:

One morning, I woke up at the rehabilitation center, and over the course of the prior evening, for some reason, I began to seriously question, "Was there seriously such a thing as heaven? Was there really an afterlife? Or when we die, are we just buried in the ground, and that's it? There's nothing else?" I was feeling intensely afraid. I was able to accept death so long as I believed there was an afterlife and Heaven, but to contemplate that there was no afterlife threatened my sanity in a way that I can't state large enough.

These are the thoughts that pervaded my mind one morning as I waited for the ambulance car to come pick me up to take me to the hospital for my radiation therapy. The ambulance soon arrived, I got in, and we left. The driver was an older man, probably in his sixties, who was quiet. As we drove, I sat in the front seat, and neither of us said anything, but after a while, he said to me, "Excuse me, but I must tell you something. I'm not quite sure how to say this, but as I'm driving here, I feel as though God is telling me that I should tell you, 'God is not going to abandon you. God is there for you now, and he will be there for you when you die.'" This guy, the ambulance car driver, spoke to me for almost half an hour as we drove to the hospital. He spoke calmly and clearly and with such specificity and credibility about the exact issue I was so very upset about. He made a definitive and very caring case that there most definitely is an afterlife, and to think otherwise is just plain wrong! He was adamant!

As he spoke, I became continuously amazed at just how specifically he kept addressing everything in my brain. It felt otherworldly. It felt as though he was reading my mind! I ended up telling him that I couldn't believe all that he was telling me because, as I explained, he was addressing the severe existential crisis I was having by thinking that, perhaps, there was no afterlife. I told him that it was so unlikely, impossible, to believe that this was a coincidence. I told him, as I sat there, I couldn't help but think that he was an angel that God sent to me to help me that day, and he told me he really couldn't explain it either, but that, as he was driving, he was overcome by the feeling that God was speaking to him and telling him to share all those things with me!

We arrived at the hospital, and he got out with me and walked me to the radiation department for my appointment. As we were both standing in front of the check-in counter, it became time for us to say goodbye, so we looked each other in the eye and said goodbye, and then we gave each other a small hug. The instant I hugged him, and I remember this shooting through my head and my heart at the time, I felt like I was a five-year-old boy hugging my father, who had passed away about ten years prior. It didn't feel like an ordinary hug; it felt like we were both clutching onto each other, holding on for dear life.

Eventually, we pushed each other apart and took a step back from one another. When I looked up at his face, he appeared to be crying, and I said, "Charlie, I love you."

And he looked intently at me, wiping his eyes, and said, "And I love you too." And that's it.

We were just about to walk away from each other when one of the hospital workers, a nice guy in his fifties, gave us a good, wise remark. He said, "Well, I don't think I've ever seen anyone say goodbye to their driver quite like that!" It was an intense, beautiful experience, and because we both felt strongly that God was speaking to us and because we told each other so, it really did feel like God was standing right there with us!

CHAPTER 13

How Not to Be a Moron

OKAY, DEAR READER, YOU HAVE ARRIVED! THIS chapter has a provocative title, but I could have also just titled this chapter, "How to Be an Effective Communicator." However, as I have already done many times in this book, I think there's a lot of value for me to share the blunt and highly effective advice that I received as I was growing up as a young boy in the 1970s. I have adjusted some of the words, and, especially in this section, I integrated my own observations.

So here's the deal: So much in life comes from one's ability to be an effective communicator. In fact, I have observed countless times, especially in my thirty-five-year career as a professional marketing communications leader, that people will often assess if someone is smart, stupid, kind, or rude simply based on how that person communicates. Hence, your communication aptitude is extremely important, so let's get started.

I'm going to start with some excellent advice that my hardworking, union-construction-working father told me. He would say, "Say what you mean and mean what you say, and do what you say you're going to do. And if you do that," he stressed, "you'll accomplish 98 percent of what's expected of you in life!" It's great advice, and it's worth adhering closely to it. Then the next pieces of advice are:

- Make sure you speak audibly. When you don't speak so people can easily hear you, it's a major problem, especially since it's such an easy problem to solve. So speak up if you have to. The next item is to be sure to acknowledge what anyone is saying to you. This, too, is extremely easy to do, which makes it all the more astonishing how many people speak too softly or at too low a volume. This whole section is about having good manners and explicitly showing respect to the other people with whom you are speaking. Think about this: What does virtually everyone speaking really want? They first want to be acknowledged. That means you're shaking your head up and down in a "yes" motion to let them know you hear them, and then people have a legitimate right to feel understood. Therefore, it's important that you motion and speak in ways that communicate that you really do understand what the speaker is saying. I know two people, in particular, who don't do these first two things: they don't acknowledge, and they offer no signs that they understand, and I can't tell you how many people have complained to me that they can't believe how rude these non-acknowledgers are, and how they no longer want to speak with them. It is so easy to acknowledge and indicate that you understand what anyone is saying, so not doing this is a way to alienate and offend people.

- I have three words in my head to describe how to be an excellent communicator and, by extension, how not to be a moron, and they are: acknowledge, understand, and affirm! We've just covered the first two: (1) Let people know you can hear them by quickly and explicitly acknowledging whoever is speaking, and then make gestures and/or say things to communicate that you understand whoever is speaking. The third trait, and you will find this is exceptionally endearing and just plain good manners, is to find a way to give the speakers affirmation of what they are saying. Importantly, you don't have to agree with whatever anyone is saying, but affirming what someone is saying is very worthy.

- You can also reflect to the speaker something positive about what the speaker is discussing. And that's it. Being affirmative is all about finding something positive to say about what the speaker has said. The great thing about this approach is when you acknowledge, understand, and affirm other people, it takes the heat off! It releases tension and puts you on a positive platform. It's no different than the advice to someone making a presentation to a large group. In that environment, the first two minutes of what you say is critical, so if you mapped out what you wanted to say and you rehearsed it so that you explicitly spoke it well, the audience feels comfortable and at ease with you, and, typically the rest of the presentation flows well because you "set it up" with intelligence and positivity, and that's just plain refreshing. If you experiment with this approach—acknowledge, understand, and affirm—I am quite confident you will begin to see just how many positive results you create. Also, it's common sense that once you make people feel comfortable and treat them with great respect, it doesn't just make for a better conversation; it opens up new doors you never even thought of. Look, just try it! If my father and his blunt-speaking male friends from the 1970s were here, they would probably say something like, "This is very easy to do, so if you can't understand it, or you won't do it, then you're a dummy." Hey, the bottom line, as I read what I just wrote, it sounds almost too simple, but, please, just give it a try. It's AUA. Remember that: "AUA!" Acknowledge, understand, and affirm.
- Now we just reviewed what you can do, but there are a few critical things that you should not do! And here they are:

1. Don't be a Negative Nelly! Reduce, if not eliminate, negativity. Stop complaining and stop saying negative things.
2. Stop contradicting. Don't be a devil's advocate: We all know people who, no matter what gets said, are con-

tradicting, always "taking issue" with what's said, or want to play "devil's advocate." It's immensely frustrating and lacks class and sophistication. It's okay to contradict or play devil's advocate once in a blue moon, but this isn't a trait you want to be known for. The last item, and this almost doesn't have to be said, is: Stop interrupting! When someone interrupts, it's like a drug. They just keep doing it more and more, and you will surely identify yourself as a moron if you frequently interrupt.

These are simple ways for anyone not to be a moron. They are all about conducting oneself with great manners and respect.

So that's it. I hope you, dear reader, find this worthwhile. I have enjoyed writing this book, and I sincerely hope you have found value in reading it. I wish you the very best in your life and all your future plans. Thank you.

David

CHAPTER 14

3 Recipes to Improve Your Life

As I HAVE TOLD YOU MY STORY, I recall one other item. The fact is that, for my entire life, I have always enjoyed cooking. My grandmother, who was from Italy, was an amazing cook, and I learned a lot from her. But also, as I met so many new people throughout my brain cancer recovery journey—another gift from God, I believe—I had the opportunity to speak with and make many new friends. As I spoke to so many new people, we would frequently start talking about food, and that would give me an opportunity to share my three favorite recipes. I would usually get their email addresses and then send these to them. I did this a lot, dozens of times! And so, I feel that it is really important—and, yes, fun(!)—to share these three recipes with you, dear reader, right now. So without further ado, here they are!

This first recipe is for *Lemon Pepper Fontina Gorgonzola Alfredo Sauce* for pasta! It's fantastic! Everyone loves it, and if you just don't like Gorgonzola blue cheese, you can substitute something else, and I make note of that below. Before we begin, as you have come to expect from me, I want to share with you a little story about where I first came by this recipe. I think it's an interesting story. You see, when I was growing up as a teenager, I worked in an exceptionally good and popular restaurant. When I was very young, perhaps sixteen years old, I was a prep cook in this very busy restaurant. The head chef was French, and he was a perfectionist who demanded that everything be perfectly cooked, and, if it ever wasn't, you'd be in a lot of trouble. One day, after I had been working there for several months and absorbing all his instructions, he said to me, "Okay, David. I've taught you a lot, and you've developed into a good cook, but now it's time for you to make your signature dish. I want you to just pluck out of your head a recipe, and I want you to cook me something right now, completely new and original. You can use any ingredients you want, just go make me something spectacular and do it right now!" And so, the honest truth is, without ever having made this before, I just made this Lemon Pepper Fontina Gorgonzola white sauce. This French chef had previously taught me how to make a Bechamel sauce, this recipe's foundation.

Here's how you do it.

In a medium-sized pot, add four tablespoons of butter and three tablespoons of olive oil. Melt the butter in the oil and stir it up. Then add two heaping tablespoons of flour and stir it up to blend it all together. Using a rubber spatula works great for this. This is commonly referred to as making a roux. You want to heat it up with the pot on medium heat and, again, stir it up well. It's okay if the flour starts to turn a golden brown, but that's it. Don't overcook it. Then add three cups of scalding hot, whole milk and stir with a whisk really fast. Blend it all together really well. You can just microwave the three cups of whole milk to get it scalding hot to pour into the roux. That's easy and a real time saver. Next, take an eight-ounce package of Fontina cheese and dice it all up into fairly small cubes. Add all of the cubed Fontina into the hot milk and roux mixture. Stir it up fast and well and just keep stirring with the pot on medium to high. You want to be careful to adjust the temperature. You want the milk to be scalding hot but no more. Be careful not to let it boil, or it will make a gigantic mess, and you will likely start crying. As soon as you start stirring the cheese in the milk, you will pretty quickly notice that you already have a smooth cheese sauce. Next, chop up two cups of soft Gorgonzola cheese and add that to your Fontina milk mixture and, again, stir it up fast and well to get it all melted and blended well together. Next, squeeze the juice of three lemons into this Fontina/Gorgonzola cheese sauce and keep stirring. Add a couple of splashes of heavy cream or about one cup. Add in a healthy amount of fresh ground pepper and just use your best judgment on how much to add. Stir, stir, stir! Now you should have a nice, smooth Lemon Pepper Fontina Gorgonzola white sauce. At this stage, take a spoon and taste a small bit of the sauce. Some people are sensitive to the taste of Gorgonzola blue cheese, so you may want to add just a little Gorgonzola at a time and keep tasting. You'll be surprised when you taste it because it's easy to tell if you want to add a little more Gorgonzola or lemon or pepper. It should be pretty close to perfect, but taste it and adjust your ingredients if you feel the need. Then cook your favorite pasta and add this on top. You can still add a little grated cheese if you'd like, and that's it! It's really very tasty!

Two more quick ideas for this sauce: If you want, you can make some penne and add a good amount of this white sauce. Then pour all that into a casserole dish and bake it in a 450-degree oven for fifteen minutes, and you'll have a fantastic mac 'n' cheese! If you really don't like blue cheese, then instead of adding Gorgonzola, just add your favorite cheese instead, and you'll get a different version of white sauce.

The last item is this white sauce also makes a fantastic white pizza. To have that, you just pour this white sauce on your pizza dough instead of using tomato sauce, then add your favorite toppings, bake in the oven, and you have a fantastic white pizza!

I have given this recipe to dozens of people and have also made it for many more. It's a real winner, and I think you will really enjoy it!

The second recipe is for *New England Style Baked Cod with a Ritz Cracker Crumb Stuffing.*

This recipe came from the restaurant I used to work at, which was located right on the ocean. This is a traditional New England way to make baked cod. It's also super easy!

Here's what you do. I'm going to give you a recipe to make one pound of cod, but you can easily make more or less just by increasing or decreasing the ingredients below.

First, melt one stick of butter. That's one-quarter pound of butter. I know that sounds like a lot, and it is. So what! If you want, use less butter, and just adjust it if you need to later!

So now you've melted one-quarter pound of butter (or a little less) in a medium-sized frying pan. To that, squeeze in the juice of half a lemon. Stir it up. Then with your hands, put about four Ritz crackers in the palm of your hand and crush them all up. It's important when you crush them that you don't want to have big pieces of crackers, and you also don't want the crackers to be crushed up so much that they turn into a powder. As the head chef used to say, "Just do it right, and don't be a moron!" With a rubber spatula, stir up and blend all the cracker crumbs into the butter and lemon. You should expect to crush up one and a half to two "sleeves" of crackers that you take from the box. Also, it's okay to buy any other brand besides Ritz, but just make sure they are like a Ritz cracker! These cracker crumbs should be fairly "wet" with butter, so just use your best judgment on whether you should add more butter or not. You're actually almost done! The final step is that you take one pound of fresh cod and spread a little olive oil on any baking pan or casserole dish and then just place the cod on top of the olive oil. Then evenly spread all the cracker crumbs over the top of the fish and tamp the crumbs down onto the top of the fish with a spatula. This stores nicely just like this in the refrigerator. When you're ready to eat, insert it into a preheated 450-degree oven for fifteen minutes, and it's done! Serve with a fresh lemon wedge.

This, too, is a fantastic meal. Serve with any vegetable or salad and, as the next recipe shows you, chicken broth-infused Basmati rice!

The third recipe is for *Chicken Broth-Infused Basmati Rice*.

The truth is, once you have white rice made with chicken broth, you'll never make it with water again!

Here's what you do:

You need a medium nonstick frying pan with a tight-fitting lid. It won't work if you don't have a good lid!

The rule is to use one part rice to three parts broth. So for example, take your favorite coffee mug and fill it up with any white rice, but I think Basmati rice is the best. Then pour that coffee cup full of rice evenly across the bottom of your nonstick medium frying pan. Then using store-bought (or homemade) chicken broth, fill that same coffee cup up three times to the same level with chicken broth, and empty the broth into the frying pan with the rice in it. You want to turn the temperature to the level where the broth will just simmer but not boil. Make sure you put the tight-fitting lid on top and let it simmer for twenty minutes. At the end of twenty minutes, all the broth should be evaporated, and the rice will be done. Just serve. It's worth noting that Bragg's Liquid Aminos soy sauce alternative is, in my opinion, light-years better tasting than regular soy sauce. This is the same brand that makes apple cider vinegar. It's really good, so give it a try, or, otherwise, use whatever soy sauce you want.

This is just a side dish for any meal, but, again, Basmati rice cooked in chicken broth is just really, really good, and you can pair this with any entrée. So give it a try and enjoy!

That's it for my recipes for you! Some people might think it's odd to include recipes in a book; however, I don't think it's odd. In fact, I think every book ought to be giving us a few good recipes, don't you think?

Maybe I'm just partial to my Italian upbringing, which was highly focused on making, having, and enjoying good food! I hope that, someday, when you make any of this food and someone asks you what it is, maybe then, you will use that as an opportunity to tell them about my book. My goal here is to create more harmony and good cheer in the world, and even if that's corny, I don't care.

I wish you bon appétit!

CHAPTER 15

Respectful

THIS IS THE FINAL CHAPTER, AND IT'S the chapter where I invite you to become an actor in my life right now.

As I said, I was diagnosed with a fatal brain cancer, however through my own assertive advocating for myself and with the Grace of God, I managed to avoid death. However, as I was undergoing radiation and chemotherapy treatments, my employer informed me that they declared bankruptcy and had to eliminate my job and all my monthly income. Because of this, I was forced to prematurely sell my beloved house and home which, ultimately bankrupted me. I then moved in with family, however it is a harsh and unhealthy environment so my story continues here where, my primary limitation these days is I don't have my own place to live, I need to buy a small home for myself, and, in this market, I conservatively estimate I need to raise $500,000 to obtain a mortgage that I can comfortably afford on my limited disability monthly income. I need some help! I have navigated the most important challenge, my life has been saved(!), but I simply need to either sell enough of this book and/or raise enough money with this fundraising link so I can afford to step into a good, strong, and positive new life.

And, so, respectfully, Dear reader, I am asking you if you will kindly make a donation to help regain my independence by raising enough money to purchase a small home for myself?

Please donate what you can reasonably afford and, Oh I have to say, if you are wealthy, please, please give me a good chunk of change, okay? And finally, if you are a billionaire, please just really help me out the best that you can.

Here's the donation weblink: https://giveahand.com/fundraiser/glioblastoma-recovery.

Thank you and God Bless you!

Authentically yours,
David Albert Francoeur

ABOUT THE AUTHOR

DAVID ALBERT FRANCOEUR IS A FIFTY-SEVEN-YEAR-OLD MAN who, since 2021, has successfully overcome fatal brain cancer, the same brain cancer that killed Senators Ted Kennedy and John McCain. In 1998, David earned distinction for being the youngest in the nation to run for U.S. Congress. While he lost that race, David was also supported by the longest-running mayor in the country. Since 1988, David spent thirty-five years climbing the corporate ladder as a C-level executive and helping to lead his employers to great success, with one becoming a "Top Ten Performer of the Decade" as cited by CNBC, and another being commended for being "At the Vanguard of Their Industry" in a front-page *Wall Street Journal* feature story.

On January 10, 2024, he authored the book *Uncommon Sense* and presents his experience and recommendations on how to assertively advocate for oneself, in this case, against a backdrop of being told he was going to die fairly soon. But then, by his unrelenting determination to challenge his doctors and to advocate exceptionally hard for himself, to the extent that one neurologist at a prominent national hospital later told him, "I think you may have just saved your own life." David Albert Francoeur's last name translates into English as "True Heart," and this book reflects both his honesty and heartfulness.

Printed in the USA
CPSIA information can be obtained
at www.ICGtesting.com
CBHW030257301024
16598CB00013B/302